Table of Contents

Introduction

If you have downloaded this book, then I am pretty sure that you have already made up your mind that you are going to walk the awesome path of the Weight Watchers Freestyle diet.

Before I go into the details of the diet though, let me talk a little bit about the origin of the program at hand.

So, the origin of the Weight Watchers diet actually goes back to the year 2912 when a humbled homemaker named Jean Nidetech (from Brooklyn), took some very strong moves in order to help obese people, which eventually led to the conception of Weight Watchers program.

Jean knows the struggles of obese people very closely, because she was an obese person herself. She went through a number of different diets and programs in order to trim down her obesity, but the Weight Watchers was the only one that allowed her to not only trim down but also keep her food hunger in check!

However, during her exploratory journey, she did take a number of different steps to trim down fat, which led to trying out a number of different diets.

This experimentation did, in fact, allow her to lose a significant amount of weight, but in doing so, she soon had an epiphany!

She soon began to realize that there are millions of people all around the world who are suffering from obesity, which inspired her to develop a solution that would help them reach their goals.

Sounds interesting right? Well, it sure is!

The Weight Watchers Freestyle is still considered as one of the most popular diet plans all around the world that is followed by millions of people.

The way how these diet works are by adding a specific amount of "SmartPoints" too food and ingredients that ultimately allows you to keep your food intake under control and encourage you to a healthier lifestyle.

The Freestyle expansion, which was established in 2017 introduced almost 200 foods that are now considered to be "Zero" points food. So, the Freestyle essentially greatly expands the array of food that you can consume without worrying about ruining your health!

Let's dive deep into the diet now and have a look at the basic concepts that make up the diet itself.

Chapter 1 The Weight Watchers Freestyle Basics

About The Program

I have already discussed this earlier, but let me elaborate on this one more time. Like I said before, unlike most of the other programs that influence you to trim down your favorite food and force you into a tight dietary shackle, the Weight Watchers in completely unique in the sense that it uses an elegantly crafted points system.

The point system allocated to the foods is further expanded and accompanied by the Physical Points system, but that won't be our focus.

You should know that the points system was previously known as "PointsPlus", which later on got upgraded to the Smart Points system that we follow today.

Somewhere around 2017, the Weight Watchers Organization took one step forward and introduced the "Freestyle Program", which brought many changes to the program, alongside the inclusion of 200 "Zero" point foods.

The core balancing act in these programs comes from how you maintain and manage your points.

Each food and ingredient have a specified SmartPoint allocated to it. Alternatively, you are allocated a specific number of weekly points based on your height, sex, weight, target weight, and various other factors.

The thing that you have to keep in mind is that you can eat as much as you want, as long as you don't exceed your allocated Smart Points limit.

Foods that are lower in Smart Points are naturally healthier and thus, safe to eat in large portions.

The Freestyle method added a few new tweaks to the formula that drastically improved the effectiveness of this program.

The Freestyle Life

Weight Watchers Freestyle allows you to eat the food that you love while losing that pesky weight! This is probably one of the core components that makes this diet so unique and awesome.

All of the foods that are allocated these "points" are very carefully studied before putting the points. The calories and various other macros are considered when the points are applied.

At the core of the process, you will be allocated a fixed number of points that you are allowed to spend over a course of the week.

Foods that are healthier sport a lower amount of points, so you can munch of healthy food as much as you can without spending your points and going overboard.

The Old SmartPoints Food List You Need to Know

Below is a list of the most common ingredients alongside their associated Smart Point for your convenience.

Food with 0 SP

- Coffee
- Banana
- Apple

- Strawberries
- Chicken Breast
- Salad
- Blueberries
- Grapes
- Tomatoes
- Watermelon
- Egg White
- Lettuce
- Deli Sliced Turkey Breast
- Baby Carrots
- Orange
- Cucumber
- Broccoli
- Water
- Green Beans
- Pineapple
- Corn on The Cob (medium)
- Cherries
- Cantaloupe
- Spinach
- Fresh Fruit
- Raspberries
- Shrimp
- Asparagus
- Celery
- Cherry Tomatoes
- Carrots
- Yogurt
- Peach
- Sweet Red Potatoes
- Pear

- Salsa
- Tuna
- Diet Coke
- Mushrooms
- Onions
- Black Beans
- Blackberries
- Zucchini
- Grape Tomatoes
- Mixed Berries
- Grapefruit
- Nectarine
- Mango
- Mustard

Food with 1 SP

- Sugar
- Almond Milk
- Egg
- Guacamole
- Half and Half
- Salad Dressing

Food with 2 SP

- Cream
- Avocado
- 1 Slice of Bread
- Scrambled Egg with milk/ butter
- Luncheon Meat, deli sliced or ham (2 ounces)
- 2 t tablespoon of Hummus

Food with 3 SP

- Milk Skimmed

- One tablespoon of Mayonnaise
- Chocolate Chip Cookies
- Sweet potatoes ½ a cup
- 3 ounces of boneless Pork Chop
- 1 ounce of flour Tortilla
- Italian Salad Dressing 2 tablespoon
- Three slices of cooked Turkey Bacon
- 1 cup of Cottage Cheese
- An ounce of crumbled Feta

Food with 4 SP

- Olive Oil
- American Cheese 1 slice
- Low Fat Milk 1%, 1 Cup
- Cheddar Cheese 1 ounce
- Red Wine 5 ounce
- ¼ cup of Almond
- 5 ounces of White Wine
- Tortilla Chips 1 ounce
- Shredded Cheddar Cheese
- One tablespoon of honey
- 102 ounces of English Muffin
- Mashed Potatoes

Food with 5 SP

- Butter
- 3 Slices of Cooked Bacon
- Reduced Fat Milk 1 Cup
- Cooked Oatmeal 1 cup
- Plain Baked Potato, 6 ounces
- Regular Beer, 12 ounces
- 1 cup of cooked regular/ whole wheat pasta
- Hamburger Bun

- Ranch Salad Dressing
- Any type of Bagel (2 ounces)
- 1 cup of Spaghetti

Food With 6+ SP

- White Rice (6)
- Brown Rice (6)
- Peanut Butter 2 tablespoon (6)
- 1 Whole Cup of Milk (7)
- 20 ounces of French Fries (13)
- 1 cup of cooked Quinoa (6)

New "0" SmartPoint Ingredients

- Peas such as chickpeas, sugar snap peas, black-eyed, etc.
- Beans such as black beans, kidney beans, pinto beans, fat-free refried beans, soybeans, sprouts, etc.
- Lentils
- Corn such as baby corn, sweet corn, corn on the cob
- Skinless Chicken Breast
- Skinless Turkey Breast
- Tofu
- Egg and Egg Whites
- Fish and Shellfish
- Yogurt
- Lean Ground Beef
- Non-Fat and Plain Greek Yogurt
- All Fruits
- All Vegetables

To give you a more detailed look at the list, the following now hold a 0 SmartPoint value.

- Yogurt
- Plain Yogurt
- Greek Yogurt

- Watermelon
- Watercress
- Water Chestnuts
- Stir Fried Vegetables
- Mixed Vegetables
- Sticks of Vegetables
- Turnips
- Turkey Breast
- Turkey Breast Tenderloin
- Ground Turkey Breast
- Tomato
- Tomato Sauce
- Tofu
- Taro
- Tangerine
- Tangelo
- Starfruit
- Winter and Summer Squash
- Spinach
- Shellfish
- Shallots
- Scallions
- Sauerkraut
- Chicken Satay
- Sashimi
- Salsa
- Salad
- Lentils
- Lime
- Lettuce
- Litchi
- Mangoes

- Mung Dal
- Mushroom Caps
- Nectarine
- Okra
- Onions
- Orange
- Parsley
- Pea Shoot
- Peaches
- Pear
- Pepper
- Pickles
- Pineapple
- Plums
- Pomegranate Seeds
- Pomelo
- Pumpkin
- Pumpkin Puree
- Radish
- Salad Mixed Greens
- Salad Three Bean
- Lemon Zest
- Leek
- Kiwifruit
- Jicama
- Jerk Chicken Breast
- Jackfruit
- Heart of Palm
- Guava
- Mixed Baby Greens
- Ginger Root
- Grape Fruit

- Fruit Cup
- Fruit Cocktail
- Fish Fillet
- Fruit
- Fish
- Figs
- Fennel
- Escarole
- Endive
- Egg Whites
- Eggs
- Apples
- Arrowroot
- Applesauce
- Artichoke
- Artichoke Hearts
- Bamboo Shoots
- Banana
- Beans
- Beets
- Blueberries
- Blackberries
- Broccoli
- Brussels
- Cabbage
- Carrots
- Cauliflower
- Cherries
- Chicken Breast
- Clementine
- Cucumber
- Dragon Fruit

- Egg Substitute
- Dates

And a few more.

Some Advantages to Know About

- Unlike most other diets, the Weight Watchers won't force you to follow an extremely restricted dietary routine
- Through the different memberships and meetings available, you will be able to get a large amount of excellent cooking advice and nutritional tips, while getting a platform to share your own experience
- Contrary to popular belief, even kids are allowed to join the program! So that they can start building up a healthy diet of their own
- The meticulously designed SmartPoints program does not only help you to lose weight but also helps to keep your food intake under control
- FitPoints (coming from various physical activities), further allows you to stay fit and healthy

Some Disadvantages to Knowing About

- While there are not glaring disadvantages of the Weight Watchers program, some individuals might feel uncomfortable when it comes to sharing their emotions in public meetings
- Keeping track of your SmartPoints might feel a little bit problematic if you are not dedicated enough
- This is a diet program that shows its true colors and effects very slowly, so one might feel discouraged while assessing the week to week progress

The Unique Changes of "Freestyle"

When considering the new Weight Watchers freestyle program, there are certain things that you should know about,

- **The new "Zero" Point foods:** This is probably the biggest change introduced in the Freestyle diet. The introduction of 200 different ingredients and foods offers you greater flexibility when creating your personalized food routine.

- **About SmartPoints:** The updated Freestyle program will still use the same method of calculation, however, your daily SmartPoint allocation will change a bit to balance out the new foods that are all zeroed out now. If you are already a member of the Weight Watchers program, then you may be able to do this with through their designated app, or alternatively, you may use the apps mentioned in the previous section.

- **Weekly Point Allowance:** Even though the allocated smart points for foods is changing, the weekly allocated points count will still be remaining the same. This essentially means that thanks to the new Points system, you will be able to consume more food within the given time.

- **Rollover Points:** This is yet another feature that is exclusive to the new program. The Rollover point system allows you to carry over a maximum of 4 SmartPoints to the coming week. So, for example, assuming that you have a weekly limit of 120 Smart Points, if you used 116 points in the previous week, you will have a SmartPoint allocation of 124 points for the upcoming week. This is a good strategy to follow if you have any major upcoming events.

And that pretty much covers the basics of the program. Now go ahead and explore the recipes!

Chapter 2 Breakfast

Hearty Pineapple Oatmeal

Serving: 5, Prep Time: 10 minutes, Cook Time: 4-8 hours

Smart Points: 7

Ingredients

- 1 cup steel cut oats
- 4 cups unsweetened almond milk
- 2 medium apples, slashed
- 1 teaspoon coconut oil
- 1 teaspoon cinnamon
- ¼ teaspoon nutmeg
- 2 tablespoons maple syrup
- A drizzle of lemon juice

Directions

1. Add listed ingredients to a cooking pan and mix well
2. Cook on very low flame for 8 hours/ or on high flame for 4 hours
3. Gently stir
4. Add toppings your desired toppings
5. Serve and enjoy!
6. Store in fridge for later use, make sure to add a splash of almond milk after re-heating for added flavor

Nutrition Values (Per Serving)

Calories: 180, Fat: 5g, Carbohydrates: 31g, Protein: 5g

Heavenly Baked Eggs

Serving: 2 , Prep Time: 5 minutes , Cook Time: 20 minutes

Smart Points: 7

Ingredients

- 2 tablespoons basil, chopped
- 2 large eggs
- 1 cup marinara sauce
- ¼ cup parmesan cheese
- Salt and pepper to taste

Directions

1. Pre-heat your oven to 350 degrees F
2. Take an oven proof skillet and pour marinara sauce, sprinkle basil
3. Make 2 cavities and break an egg into the cavities, sprinkle cheese, pepper
4. Place in your oven in the middle rack and bake for 20 minutes
5. Serve and enjoy!

Nutrition Values (Per Serving)

Calories: 180 , Fat: 5g , Carbohydrates: 31g , Protein: 5g

Wholesome Pumpkin Pie Oatmeal

Serving: 2 , Prep Time: 10 minutes , Cook Time: 10 minutes

Smart Points: 6

Ingredients

- ½ cup canned pumpkin
- Mashed banana as needed
- ¾ cup unsweetened almond milk
- ½ teaspoon pumpkin pie spice
- 1 cup oats
- 2 teaspoons maple syrup

Directions

1. Mash banana using fork and mix in the remaining ingredients (except oats) and mix well
2. Add oats and finely stir
3. Transfer mixture to a pot and let the oats cook until it has absorbed the liquid and are tender
4. Serve and enjoy!

Nutrition Values (Per Serving)

Calories: 264 , Fat: 4g , Carbohydrates: 52g , Protein: 7g

Classic Eggs in Muffin Tin

Serving: 6 , Prep Time: 10 minutes , Cook Time: 30 minutes

Smart Points: 0

Ingredients

- ½ teaspoon sage
- ½ teaspoon pepper
- ¼ teaspoon red pepper flakes
- ½ pound ground turkey
- 1 bell pepper, diced
- 12 whole eggs
- ¼ teaspoon salt
- ¼ teaspoon Marjoram

Directions

1. Pre-heat your oven to 350 degrees F
2. Grease a cupcake tin with non-stick spray
3. Take a skillet and place it over medium heat, add turkey and cook
4. Beat in eggs with seasoning, stir in bell pepper and cooked turkey to the egg mixture
5. Divide egg mixture between muffin tins and bake for 30 minutes
6. Once the eggs are set, enjoy!

Nutrition Values (Per Serving)

Calories: 172 , Fat: 10g , Carbohydrates: 2g , Protein: 16g

Best Egg and Avocado Toast in A Hole

Serving: 2, Prep Time: 10 minutes, Cook Time: 10 minutes

Smart Points: 6

Ingredients

- 2 and ½ slices whole wheat bread
- Olive oil spray
- Fresh ground pepper
- Hot sauce to taste
- Salt to taste
- 2 and ½ ounces avocado flesh, mashed
- 2 large eggs

Directions

1. Take your bread slices and make a hole in the middle using a cookie cutter
2. Season avocado mash with salt and pepper
3. Take a skillet and place it over medium-low heat, grease with cooking spray
4. Place bread slices and a cut portion in the skillet
5. Break egg into the hole of the bread, cook until the egg properly settles down, season with more salt and pepper
6. Flip and cook the other side
7. Once done, transfer to a plate
8. Top the egg with avocado mash, hot sauce and crumble bread (made from the cut piece)
9. Enjoy!

Nutrition Values (Per Serving)

Calories: 229 , Fat: 23g , Carbohydrates: 10g , Protein: 12g

Eggy Tomato Scramble

Serving: 2, Prep Time: 10 minutes, Cook Time: 5 minutes

Smart Points: 4

Ingredients

- 8 whole eggs
- ½ cup fresh basil, chopped
- 2 tablespoons olive oil
- ½ teaspoon red pepper flakes, crushed
- 1 cup grape tomatoes, chopped
- Salt and pepper to taste

Directions

1. Take a bowl and whisk in eggs, salt, pepper, red pepper flakes and mix well
2. Add tomatoes, basil, and mix
3. Take a skillet and place it over medium-high heat
4. Add egg mixture and cook for 5 minutes and cooked and scrambled
5. Enjoy!

Nutrition Values (Per Serving)

Calories: 130 , Fat: 10g , Carbohydrates: 8g , Protein: 1.8g

Fresh Early Morning Pineapple Juice

Serving: 2 , Prep Time: 10 minutes , Cook Time: Nil

Smart Points: 3

Ingredients

- 4 cups fresh pineapple, chopped
- 1 pinch salt
- 1 and ½ cup of water

Directions

1. Add listed ingredients to blender and pulse until smooth
2. Strain juice through a strainer and serve in 3 glasses, chilled
3. Enjoy!

Nutrition Values (Per Serving)

Calories: 82 , Fat: 0.2g , Carbohydrates: 0.9g , Protein: 21g

Classical Pancakes

Serving: 4 , Prep Time: 10 minutes , Cook Time: 5 minutes

Smart Points: 1

Ingredients

- 1 teaspoon salt
- ½ cup low-fat milk
- 1 cup all-purpose flour
- 1 teaspoon vanilla
- 4 beaten eggs
- 1 teaspoon baking soda
- 2 cups non-fat Greek yogurt

Directions

1. Add Greek yogurt to your bowl and mix in the dry ingredients in another bowl
2. Stir the mixture into your yogurt and make sure everything is mixed well
3. Stir in eggs, milk, vanilla and stir well
4. Stir the mixture into the yogurt batter and add more flour to thicken it up
5. Take a skillet and place it over medium heat, add pancake batter and cook until bubbles appear
6. Flip and cook the other side
7. Repeat with remaining batter and enjoy!

Nutrition Values (Per Serving)

Calorie: 212 , Fat: 2g , Carbohydrates: 28g , Protein: 2g

Decisive Egg Salad

Serving: 4 , Prep Time: 5 minutes , Cook Time: 10 minutes

Smart Points: 5

Ingredients

- ¼ teaspoon pepper
- ½ teaspoon salt
- 1-piece dill
- 2 tablespoons mayonnaise
- ½ teaspoon Dijon mustard
- 2 tablespoons chives
- 4 whole eggs
- 2 hardboiled eggs

Directions

1. Take a pan and fill it with water, add eggs and place on high heat
2. Bring to a boil
3. Once eggs are done, drain water and add eggs to ice water bath
4. Once cooled, remove shells
5. Gently remove yolks from two eggs and slice them up
6. Add pepper, salt, mustard, dill, chives, and mayo to a bowl and stir well, add sliced up egg whites and egg yolks
7. Mix well
8. Enjoy!

Nutrition Values (Per Serving)

Calories: 298 , Fat: 4g , Carbohydrates: 55g , Protein: 11g

Awesome Breakfast Parfait

Serving: 2 , Prep Time: 5 minutes , Cook Time: Nil

Smart Points: 1

Ingredients

- 1 teaspoon salt
- ½ cup low-fat milk
- 1 cup all-purpose flour
- 1 teaspoon vanilla
- 4 beaten eggs
- 1 teaspoon baking soda
- 2 cups non-fat Greek yogurt

Directions

1. Break up pretzels into small sized portions and slice up the strawberries
2. Add yogurt to the bottom of the glass and top with pretzels pieces and strawberries
3. Add more yogurt and keep repeating until you have used up all ingredients
4. Enjoy!

Nutrition Values (Per Serving)

Calorie: 304 , Fat: 1g , Carbohydrates: 58g , Protein: 15g

Chapter 3 Beef and Pork

Juicy and Peppery Tenderloin

Serving: 4 ,Prep Time: 10 minutes , Cook Time: 20

Smart Points: 4

Ingredients

- 2 teaspoons sage, chopped
- Salt and pepper
- 2 and1/2 pounds beef tenderloin
- 2 teaspoon thyme, chopped
- 2 garlic cloves, sliced
- 2 teaspoons rosemary, chopped
- 4 teaspoons olive oil

Directions

1. Pre-heat your oven to 425 degrees F
2. Take a small knife and cut incisions on tenderloin, insert one slice of garlic into the incision
3. Rub meat with oil
4. Take a bowl and add salt, sage, thyme, rosemary, pepper and mix well
5. Rub spice mix over tenderloin
6. Put rubbed tenderloin into roasting pan and bake for 10 minutes
7. Lower temperature to 350 degrees F and cooks for 20 minutes more until an internal thermometer reads 145 degrees F
8. Transfer tenderloin to cutting board and let them sit for 15 minutes, slice into 20 pieces and enjoy!

Nutrition Values (Per Serving)

Calorie: 183 , Fat: 9g , Carbohydrates: 1g , Protein: 24g

South-Western Pork Chops

Serving: 4 , Prep Time: 10 minutes , Cook Time: 15 minutes

Smart Points: 3

Ingredients

- Cooking spray as needed
- 4-ounce pork loin chop, boneless and fat rimmed
- 1/3 cup of salsa
- 2 tablespoon of fresh lime juice
- ¼ cup of fresh cilantro, chopped

Directions

1. Take a large sized non-stick skillet and spray it with cooking spray
2. Heat it up until hot over high eat
3. Press the chops with your palm to flatten them slightly
4. Add them to the skillet and cook on 1 minute for each side until they are nicely browned
5. Lower down the heat to medium-low
6. Combine the salsa and lime juice
7. Pour the mix over the chops
8. Simmer uncovered for about 8 minutes until the chops are perfectly done
9. If needed, sprinkle some cilantro on top
10. Serve!

Nutrition Values (Per Serving)

Calorie: 184 , Fat: 4g , Carbohydrates: 4g , Protein: 0.5g

The Original BBQ Meatloaf

Serving: 3, Prep Time: 5 minutes, Cook Time: 40 minutes

Smart Points: 6

Ingredients

- 1 pound 93% lean ground beef
- ½ a cup of BBQ sauce
- ¼ cup of frozen chopped onion pressed dry
- ¼ cup of seasoned Italian bread crumbs
- 2 large egg whites

Directions

1. Pre-heat your oven to 375 degrees F
2. Take a bowl and add meat, ¼ cup of BBQ sauce, onion, egg whites, bread crumbs, seasoning of your choice
3. Stir
4. Shape the mixture into a loaf pan
5. Spread remaining ¼ cup of BBQ sauce over loaf
6. Bake for 40 minutes at 375 degrees Fahrenheit
7. Check the doneness and enjoy!

Nutrition Values (Per Serving)

Calorie: 240 , Fat: 6g , Carbohydrates: 17g , Protein: 27g

Caramelized Pork Chops and Onion

Serving: 4 , Prep Time: 5 minutes , Cook Time: 40 minutes

Smart Points: 3

Ingredients

- 4-pound chuck roast
- 4-ounce green Chili, chopped
- 2 tablespoon of chili powder
- ½ a teaspoon of dried oregano
- ½ a teaspoon of cumin, ground
- 2 garlic cloves, minced
- Salt as needed

Directions

1. Rub the chops with a seasoning of 1 teaspoon of pepper and 2 teaspoons of salt
2. Take a skillet and place it over medium heat, add oil and allow the oil to heat up
3. Brown the seasoned chop both sides
4. Add water and onion to the skillet and cover, lower down the heat to low and simmer for 20 minutes
5. Turn the chops over and season with more salt and pepper
6. Cover and cook until the water fully evaporates and the beer shows a slightly brown texture
7. Remove the chops and serve with a topping of the caramelized onion
8. Serve and enjoy!

Nutrition Values (Per Serving)

Calorie: 47 , Fat: 4g , Carbohydrates: 4g , Protein: 0.5g

Spiced Up Organic Meatball

Serving: 4 , Prep Time: 10 minutes , Cook Time: 25 minutes + 2-4 hours

Smart Points: 8

Ingredients

- 2 whole eggs
- 2 pounds organic beef, ground
- 4-5 tablespoons fruit-sweetened grape jelly
- 1/2 teaspoon pepper, ground
- ½ teaspoon Spanish paprika
- ¼ teaspoon chili powder
- 1 teaspoon ground garlic salt
- ¼ cup tapioca flour

Directions

1. Pre-heat your oven to 350 degrees F
2. Add beef, pepper, eggs, garlic, salt, tapioca starch in a bowl
3. Mix well and make balls
4. Transfer to a baking sheet
5. Bake for 25 minutes
6. Transfer to a pot and add chili sauce, paprika, grape jelly, and chili powder
7. Cook on very flame for 2-4 hours (use a crockpot if possible)
8. Enjoy!

Nutrition Values (Per Serving)

Calories: 288 , Carbohydrates: 34g , Protein: 2g

Fascinating Spinach and Beef Meatballs

Serving: 4 , Prep Time: 10 minutes , Cook Time: 20

Smart Points: 4

Ingredients

- ½ cup onion
- 4 garlic cloves
- 1 whole egg
- ¼ teaspoon oregano
- Salt and pepper to taste
- 1-pound lean ground beef
- 10 ounces spinach

Directions

1. Pre-heat your oven to 375 degrees F
2. Take a bowl and mix in the rest of the ingredients, mix using your hands and roll into meatballs
3. Transfer to a sheet tray and bake for 20 minutes
4. Enjoy!

Nutrition Values (Per Serving)

Calorie: 200 , Fat: 8g , Carbohydrates: 5g , Protein: 29g

Lovely Mongolian Beef

Serving: 4 , Prep Time: 10 minutes , Cook Time: 20

Smart Points: 4

Ingredients

- 2 teaspoons Asian garlic chili paste
- 2 teaspoons vegetable oil
- 1 tablespoon rice vinegar
- 1-pound sirloin beef, lean and cubed
- 16 green onions, chopped
- 1 tablespoon ginger minced
- 2 tablespoons low soy sauce
- 1 garlic clove, minced
- 1 teaspoon cornstarch
- 1 tablespoon hoisin sauce

Directions

1. Take a bowl and stir in soy sauce, cornstarch, hoisin sauce, rice vinegar, chili paste
2. Add ginger, garlic, beef to a heated skillet and Saute for 3 minutes until the beef is nice and golden
3. Mix in sauce, green onions and cook for a few minutes
4. Enjoy!

Nutrition Values (Per Serving)

Calorie: 231 , Fat: 7g , Carbohydrates: 10g , Protein: 27g

Generously Smothered Pork Chops

Serving: 4, Prep Time: 10 minutes , Cook Time: 30 minutes

Smart Points: 6

Ingredients

- 4 pork chops, bone-in
- 2 tablespoon of olive oil
- ¼ cup of vegetable broth
- ½ a pound of Yukon gold potatoes, peeled and chopped
- 1 large onion, sliced
- 2 garlic cloves, minced
- 2 teaspoons of rubbed sage
- 1 teaspoon of thyme, ground
- Salt and pepper as needed

Directions

1. Pre-heat your oven to 350 degrees Fahrenheit
2. Take a large sized skillet and place it over medium heat
3. Add a tablespoon of oil and allow the oil to heat up
4. Add pork chops and cook them for 4-5 minutes per side until browned
5. Transfer chops to a baking dish
6. Pour broth over the chops
7. Add remaining oil to the pan and Sauté potatoes, onion, garlic for 3-4 minutes
8. Take a large bowl and add potatoes, garlic, onion, thyme, sage, pepper, and salt
9. Transfer this mixture to the baking dish (wish pork)
10. Bake for 20-30 minutes
11. Serve and enjoy!

Nutrition Values (Per Serving)

Calorie: 261, Fat: 10g, Carbohydrates: 1.3g, Protein: 2g

Chapter 4 Poultry

Cool Chicken Burrito Bowl

Serving: 4, Prep Time: 5 minutes, Cook Time: 25-30

Smart Points: 6

Ingredients

- Salt and pepper as needed
- 1-pound skinless chicken breast
- 1 can black beans
- 1 teaspoon garlic powder
- ½ onion, sliced
- 1 can fire roasted tomatoes
- 2 bell peppers, sliced
- 1 tablespoon olive oil
- 1 teaspoon cumin
- ½ teaspoon paprika
- 1 and ½ cups low sodium chicken broth
- 2 teaspoons chili powder
- ½ teaspoon oregano

Directions

1. Take a bowl and mix in chili powder, garlic powder, oregano, salt, pepper, paprika and cumin
2. Add chicken in half of the spice mix and pan fry for 5 minutes (each side)
3. After the chicken is done, mix in peppers and onions, cook for 5 minutes more
4. Stir in black beans, tomatoes, chicken broth, rice
5. Turn heat to low and bring to simmer, cook for 25 minutes
6. Enjoy!

Nutrition Values (Per Serving)

Calorie: 496, Fat: 6g, Carbohydrates: 66g, Protein: 37g

Fantastic Grilled BBQ Chicken

Serving: 4 , Prep Time: 5 minutes , Cook Time: 30-40

Smart Points: 4

Ingredients

- 1 teaspoon sriracha
- 1 teaspoon ginger, minced
- ¼ cup pineapple juice
- 2 tablespoons soy sauce
- The ½ cup BBQ sauce
- 1 teaspoon garlic, minced
- 2 cups pineapple, sliced

Directions

1. Take a bowl and stir in garlic, sriracha, soy sauce, garlic, BBQ, pineapple juice and mix well
2. Add chicken and let it marinate for 30 minutes
3. Grill pineapple slices and chicken in hot pan, cook until the internal temperature reaches 165 degrees F and the pineapple are finely caramelized
4. Bring leftover marinade to boil and serve pineapple with chicken and extra sauce
5. Enjoy!

Nutrition Values (Per Serving)

Calorie: 270 , Fat: 2g , Carbohydrates: 25g , Protein: 33g

Berry Flavored Balsamic Chicken

Serving: 4, Prep Time: 10 minutes, Cook Time: 35 minutes

Smart Points: 3

Ingredients

- 3 boneless chicken breasts, skinless
- Salt and pepper as needed
- ¼ cup of all-purpose flour
- 2/3 cup of low-fat chicken broth
- 1 and a ½ teaspoon of corn starch
- ½ a cup of low sugar raspberry preserve
- 1 and a ½ tablespoon of balsamic vinegar

Directions

1. Cut the chicken breast into bite-sized portions and season with salt and pepper
2. Dredge the meat in flour and shake off any excess
3. Take a non-stick skillet and place it over medium heat
4. Add chicken and cook for 15 minutes, making sure to turn once halfway through
5. Remove chicken and transfer to a platter
6. Add cornstarch, broth, raspberry preserve into the same skillet and stir
7. Stir in balsamic vinegar and keep the heat on medium, stir cook for a few minutes
8. Transfer the chicken back to the skillet and cook for 15 minutes more, turning once
9. Serve and enjoy!

Nutrition Values (Per Serving)

Calorie: 546, Fat: 35g, Carbohydrates: 25g, Protein: 33g

Stir Fried Chicken Dish

Serving: 4, Prep Time: 20 minutes, Cook Time: 25 minutes

Smart Points: 5

Ingredients

- 2 and a ½ pounds of skinless, boneless chicken breast, sliced thin
- 4 tablespoon of fish sauce
- 2 teaspoons of Swerve
- 2 onions, thinly sliced
- 8 scallions, sliced
- ½ a cup of fresh cilantro, chopped
- 4 tablespoon of soy sauce
- 2 tablespoon of chili garlic sauce
- 4 tablespoon of olive oil
- 4 garlic cloves, minced
- Salt and pepper as needed

Directions

1. Take a bowl and add fish sauce, swerve, soy sauce and chili garlic sauce and mix well
2. Dredge the chicken in your sauce mixture and let it marinate for 10 minutes
3. Take a large skillet and place it over medium-high heat
4. Add oil and allow the oil to heat up
5. Add onions and Sauté for 4 minutes, add garlic and Sauté for 1 minute more
6. Add chicken and marinade and Sauté for 7 minutes
7. Add cilantro and scallions
8. Cook for 3 minutes more and stir in basil
9. Cook for 1 minute

10. Season with salt and pepper
11. Stir and enjoy!

Nutrition Values (Per Serving)

Calorie: 229, Fat: 8g, Carbohydrates: 10g, Protein: 29g

Delicious Thai Garlic Chicken

Serving: 4, Prep Time: 10 minutes, Cook Time: 5 minutes

Smart Points: 6

Ingredients

- 1-pound chicken breast tenders
- Cooking spray as needed
- ¼ cup garlic chili sauce
- 2 tablespoons honey
- 1 teaspoon salt
- 1 teaspoon pepper
- 2 cups asparagus spears, chopped
- 1 cup onion, sliced
- 1 tablespoon olive oil
- Cooked rice for serving

Directions

1. Pre-heat your oven to 375 degrees F
2. Spray 8x8 baking dish with cooking spray
3. Place chicken in single layer in baking dish, season with salt and pepper
4. Take a bowl and add garlic chili sauce, honey, and mix well
5. Pour sauce mixture over chicken, add asparagus and onion
6. Drizzle olive oil
7. Bake for 25-30 minutes
8. Remove from oven and let it rest
9. Enjoy!

Nutrition Values (Per Serving)

Calories: 242, Fat: 4g, Carbohydrates: 17g, Protein: 28g

Hearty Chicken Fried Rice

Serving: 4 , Prep Time: 10 minutes , Cook Time: 12 minutes

Smart Points: 2

Ingredients

- 1 teaspoon olive oil
- 4 large egg whites
- 1 onion, chopped
- 2 garlic cloves, minced
- 12 ounces skinless chicken breasts, boneless, cut into ½ inch cubes
- ½ cup carrots, chopped
- ½ cup of frozen green peas
- 2 cups long grain brown rice, cooked
- 3 tablespoons soy sauce, low sodium

Directions

1. Coat skillet with oil, place it over medium-high heat
2. Add egg whites and cook until scrambled
3. Sauté onion, garlic and chicken breasts for 6 minutes
4. Add carrots, peas and keep cooking for 3 minutes
5. Stir in rice, season with soy sauce
6. Add cooked egg whites, stir for 3 minutes
7. Enjoy!

Nutrition Values (Per Serving)

Calories: 353 , Fat: 11g , Carbohydrates: 30g , Protein: 23g

Hearty Lemon and Pepper Chicken

Serving: 4, Prep Time: 5 minutes, Cook Time: 15

Smart Points: 3

Ingredients

- 2 teaspoons olive oil
- 1 and ¼ pounds skinless chicken cutlets
- 2 whole eggs
- ¼ cup panko
- 1 tablespoon lemon pepper
- Salt and pepper to taste
- 3 cups green beans
- ¼ cup parmesan cheese
- ¼ teaspoon garlic powder

Directions

1. Pre-heat your oven to 425 degrees F
2. Take a bowl and stir in seasoning, parmesan, lemon pepper, garlic powder, panko
3. Whisk eggs in another bowl
4. Coat cutlets in eggs and press into panko mix
5. Transfer coated chicken to a parchment lined a baking sheet
6. Toss the beans in oil, pepper, and salt, lay them on the side of the baking sheet
7. Bake for 15 minutes
8. Enjoy!

Nutrition Values (Per Serving)

Calorie: 299 , Fat: 10g , Carbohydrates: 10g , Protein: 43g

Tiny Buffalo Chicken Bites

Serving: 4 , Prep Time: 10 minutes , Cook Time: 12 minutes

Smart Points: 3

Ingredients

- 4 ounces fat cream cheese
- 1 tablespoon cayenne sauce
- 10 ounces tomatoes, diced
- 5 ounces chicken, chunks
- ½ cup reduced fat cheddar cheese, shredded
- 22 frozen mini filo shells
- 1 stalk celery

Directions

1. Pre-heat your stove to 350 degrees F
2. Place cream cheddar and pepper sauce in medium microwave-safe bowl
3. Microwave on HIGH for 30 seconds
4. Add depleted tomatoes, chicken, cheddar, stir well
5. Partition the blend into your shells and bake for 8-12 minutes
6. Serve and enjoy!

Nutrition Values (Per Serving)

Calories: 75 , Fat: 5g , Carbohydrates: 5g , Protein: 4g

Amazing Grilled Chicken and Blueberry Salad

Serving: 5 , Prep Time: 10 minutes , Cook Time: 25 minutes

Smart Points: 9

Ingredients

- 5 cups mixed greens
- 1 cup blueberries
- ¼ cup slivered almonds
- 2 cups chicken breasts, cooked and cubed

For dressing

- ¼ cup olive oil
- ¼ cup apple cider vinegar
- ¼ cup blueberries
- 2 tablespoons honey
- Salt and pepper to taste

Directions

1. Take a bowl and add greens, berries, almonds, chicken cubes and mix well
2. Take a bowl and mix the dressing ingredients, pour the mix into a blender and blitz until smooth
3. Add dressing on top of the chicken cubes and toss well
4. Season more and enjoy!

Nutrition Values (Per Serving)

Calories: 266 , Fat: 17g , Carbohydrates: 18g , Protein: 10g

Chapter 5 Vegetarian Recipes

The Garbanzo Bean Extravaganza

Serving: 5 , Prep Time: 10 minutes , Cook Time: Nil

Smart Points: 5

Ingredients

- 1 can garbanzo beans, chickpeas
- 1 tablespoon olive oil
- 1 teaspoon salt
- 1 teaspoon garlic powder
- ½ teaspoon paprika

Directions

1. Pre-heat your oven to 375 degrees F
2. Line a baking sheet with silicone baking mat
3. Drain and rinse garbanzo beans, pat garbanzo beans dry and pout into a large bowl
4. Toss with olive oil, salt, garlic powder, paprika and mix well
5. Spread over a baking sheet
6. Bake for 20 minutes at 375 degrees F
7. Turn chickpeas so they are roasted well
8. Place back in oven and bake for 25 minutes at 375 degrees F
9. Let them cool and enjoy!

Nutrition Values (Per Serving)

Calories: 395 , Fat: 7g , Carbohydrates: 52g , Protein: 35g

Apple Slices

Serving: 4 , Prep Time: 10 minutes , Cook Time: 10 minutes

Smart Points: 1

Ingredients

- 1 cup of coconut oil
- ¼ cup date paste
- 2 tablespoons ground cinnamon
- 4 granny smith apples, peeled and sliced, cored

Directions

1. Take a large sized skillet and place it over medium heat
2. Add oil and allow the oil to heat up
3. Stir in cinnamon and date paste into the oil
4. Add cut up apples and cook for 5-8 minutes until crispy
5. Serve and enjoy!

Nutrition Values (Per Serving)

Calories: 368 , Fat: 23g , Carbohydrates: 44g , Protein: 1g

Authentic Zucchini Boats

Serving: 4 , Prep Time: 10 minutes , Cook Time: 25 minutes

Smart Points: 3

Ingredients

- 4 medium zucchinis
- ½ cup marinara sauce
- ¼ red onion, sliced
- ¼ cup kalamata olives, chopped
- ½ cup cherry tomatoes, sliced
- 2 tablespoons fresh basil

Directions

1. Pre-heat your oven to 400 degrees Fahrenheit
2. Cut the zucchini half-lengthwise and shape them in boats
3. Take a bowl and add tomato sauce, spread 1 layer of sauce on top of each of the boat
4. Top with onion, olives, and tomatoes
5. Bake for 20-25 minutes
6. Top with basil and enjoy!

Nutrition Values (Per Serving)

Calories: 278 , Fat: 20g , Carbohydrates: 10g , Protein: 15g

Grilled Sprouts and Balsamic Glaze

Serving: 2 , Prep Time: 10 minutes , Cook Time: 30 minutes

Smart Points: 4

Ingredients

- ½ pound Brussels sprouts, trimmed and halved
- Fresh cracked black pepper
- 1 tablespoon olive oil
- Salt to taste
- 2 teaspoons balsamic glaze
- 2 wooden skewers

Directions

1. Take wooden skewers and place them on a largely sized foil
2. Place sprouts on the skewers and drizzle oil sprinkle salt and pepper
3. Cover skewers with foil
4. Pre-heat your grill to low and place skewers (with foil) in the grill
5. Grill for 30 minutes, making sure to turn after every 5-6 minutes
6. Once done, uncovered and drizzle balsamic glaze on top
7. Enjoy!

Nutrition Values (Per Serving)

Calories: 440 , Fat: 27g , Carbohydrates: 33g , Protein: 26g

Delicious Pesto Parm Baked Tomatoes

Serving: 4 , Prep Time: 5 minutes , Cook Time: 5 minutes

Smart Points: 1

Ingredients

- 2 tomatoes, halved
- 3 tablespoons parmesan cheese, shredded
- 2 teaspoons basil pesto

Directions

1. Add tomatoes, with cut side up on a baking sheet
2. Spread ½ teaspoon pesto over each tomato half, sprinkle cheese
3. Broil in preheated broil for 4-5 minutes until cheese melts
4. Serve and enjoy!

Nutrition Values (Per Serving)

Calories: 354 , Fat: 1g , Carbohydrates: 45g , Protein: 0.2g

Simple Creamy Pesto Pasta

Serving: 4 , Prep Time: 10 minutes , Cook Time: 10 minutes

Smart Points: 5

Ingredients

- 1 teaspoon lemon juice
- 1 and ½ teaspoon olive oil
- 2 and ½ tablespoons cream cheese
- 2 garlic cloves
- 4 and ½ cups baby spinach
- 2 tablespoons water
- 1 and ¼ teaspoon salt
- 8 ounces spaghetti, uncooked

Directions

1. Take a pot and add water, bring to a boil
2. Add a little bit of salt and add pasta, cook for 8 minutes
3. Drain water and top with cherry tomatoes, parmesan cheese
4. Add salt, oil, garlic, spinach, and water to a blender and mix well
5. Add cream cheese to pasta and stir until melts
6. Add water and pesto sauce until you have the right consistency
7. Season with lemon juice and enjoy!

Nutrition Values (Per Serving)

Calories: 288 , Fat: 5g , Carbohydrates: 34g , Protein: 2g

A Turtle Friend Salad

Serving: 6 , Prep Time: 5 minutes , Cook Time: 5 minutes

SmartPoints: 1

Ingredients

- 1 Romaine lettuce, chopped
- 3 Roma tomatoes, diced
- 1 English cucumber, diced
- 1 small red onion, diced
- ½ cup parsley, chopped
- 2 tablespoons virgin olive oil
- ½ large lemon, juice
- 1 teaspoon garlic powder
- Salt and pepper to taste

Directions

1. Wash the vegetables thoroughly under cold water
2. Prepare them by chopping, dicing or mincing as needed
3. Take a large salad bowl and transfer the prepped veggies
4. Add vegetable oil, olive oil, lemon juice, and spice
5. Toss well to coat
6. Serve chilled if preferred
7. Enjoy!

Nutrition Values (Per Serving)

Calories: 200 , Fat: 8g , Carbohydrates: 18g , Protein: 10g

Exceptional Watercress and Melon Salad

Serving: 4 , Prep Time: 15 minutes , Cook Time: 20 minutes

SmartPoints: 1

Ingredients

- 3 tablespoons lime juice
- 1 teaspoon date paste
- 1 teaspoon fresh ginger root, minced
- ¼ cup of vegetable oil
- 2 bunch watercress, chopped
- 2 and ½ cups watermelon, cubed
- 2 and ½ cups cantaloupe, cubed
- 1/3 cup almonds, toasted and sliced

Directions

1. Take a large sized bowl and add lime juice, ginger, date paste
2. Whisk well and add oil
3. Season with pepper and salt
4. Add watercress, watermelon
5. Toss well
6. Transfer to a serving bowl and garnish with sliced almonds
7. Enjoy!

Nutrition Values (Per Serving)

Calories: 274 , Fat: 20g , Carbohydrates: 21g , Protein: 7g

Chapter 6 Soups and Stews

Broccoli and Cheese Delight

Serving: 2 , Prep Time: 10 minutes , Cook Time: 35 minutes

SmartPoints: 3

Ingredients

- 3 can of 14 and ½ ounce (each) chicken broth
- 2 bag (1 pound each) frozen broccoli
- 1 can of 10 and a ½ ounce (each) tomatoes and green chili pepper
- 10-ounce Velveeta low-fat cheese

Directions

1. Take a pot and add broth, frozen broccoli, tomatoes and chili
2. Mix well and place it over medium-high heat
3. Allow the mixture to heat up and reach a boil
4. Lower down the heat to low and simmer for 25 minutes until the veggies are tender
5. Cube Velveeta and drop them into the soup
6. Simmer until the cheese melts
7. Serve and enjoy!

Nutrition Values (Per Serving)

Calories: 112 , Fat: 4g , Carbohydrates: 9g , Protein: 11g

Ideal Potato Soup

Serving: 4-6 , Prep Time: 5 minutes , Cook Time: 28 minutes

SmartPoints:2

Ingredients

- 2 tablespoons extra virgin olive oil
- 1 large sized onion, chopped
- 2 garlic cloves, crushed
- 1-pound sweet potato, peeled and cut into medium pieces
- ½ teaspoon ground cumin
- ¼ teaspoon ground chili
- ½ teaspoon ground coriander
- ¼ teaspoon ground cinnamon
- ¼ teaspoon salt
- 2 cups chicken stock
- Low-fat crème Fraiche
- Fresh parsley, chopped
- Coriander as needed

Directions

1. Take a large sized pan and place it over medium-high heat
2. Add olive oil and heat it up
3. Add onions and Sauté them until they are slightly browned
4. Turn down the heat to medium and add garlic and keep cooking for 2-3 minutes more
5. Add sweet potato and Sauté for 3-4 minutes
6. Add the remaining spices and season with some salt
7. Cook for 2 minutes
8. Pour stock and turn the heat up
9. Bring the mixture to a boil and give it a stir

10. Put a lid on top and lower down the lid and bring it to a slow simmer
11. Cook for 20 minutes until the potatoes are tender
12. Remove the pan from the heat
13. Take an immersion blender and puree the whole mixture
14. Add a bit of water if the soup is too thick
15. Check the soup for seasoning
16. Ladle the soup into your serving bowls
17. Give a swirl of crème Fraiche
18. Sprinkle some chopped up parsley
19. Enjoy!

Nutrition Values (Per Serving)

Calories: 324 , Fat: 7g , Carbohydrates: 25g , Protein: 12g

Greek Lemon and Chicken Soup

Serving: 4 , Prep Time: 15 minutes , Cook Time: 30 minutes

SmartPoints: 2

Ingredients

- 2 cups cooked chicken, chopped
- 2 medium carrots, chopped
- ½ a cup of onion, chopped
- ¼ cup lemon juice
- 1 clove garlic, minced
- 1 can cream of chicken soup, fat-free and low sodium
- 2 cans of chicken broth, fat-free
- ¼ teaspoon of ground black pepper
- 2/3 cup of long-grain rice
- 2 tablespoons of parsley, snipped

Directions

1. Add all of the listed ingredients to a pot (except rice and parsley)
2. Season with salt and pepper
3. Bring the mix to a boil over medium-high heat
4. Stir in rice and set heat to medium
5. Simmer for 20 minutes until rice is tender
6. Garnish parsley and enjoy!

Nutrition Values (Per Serving)

Calories: 582 , Fat: 33g , Carbohydrates: 35g , Protein: 32g

Awesome Egg Drop Soup

Serving: 5 , Prep Time: 5 minutes , Cook Time: 5 minutes

SmartPoints: 1

Ingredients

- 4 cups low sodium chicken broth
- ½ teaspoon soy sauce
- ½ cup chicken breast, cooked, boneless and skinless
- ½ cup of frozen green peas
- ¼ cup green onions, sliced
- 1 egg, lightly beaten

Directions

1. Take a saucepan and place it over medium heat, add chicken stock and soy sauce
2. Bring the mix to a boil and add peas, green onions chicken and stir
3. Bring the mix to boil once again
4. Remove the heat and slowly drizzle in the egg
5. Wait for a minute until the egg sets in
6. Stir and ladle the soup into serving bowls
7. Enjoy!

Nutrition Values (Per Serving)

Calories: 119 , Fat: 4g , Carbohydrates: 8g , Protein: 14g

Awesome Cabbage Soup

Serving: 3 , Prep Time: 7 minutes, Cook Time: 25 minutes

SmartPoints: 1

Ingredients

- 3 cups non-fat beef stock
- 2 garlic cloves, minced
- 1 tablespoon of tomato paste
- 2 cup cabbage, chopped
- ½ a yellow onion
- ½ a cup carrot, chopped
- ½ a cup green bean
- ½ a cup zucchini, chopped
- ½ a teaspoon of basil
- ½ a teaspoon of oregano
- Salt and pepper as needed

Directions

1. Grease a pot with non-stick cooking spray
2. Place it over medium heat and allow the oil the heat up
3. Add onions, carrots, and garlic and Sauté for 5 minutes
4. Add broth, tomato paste, green beans, cabbage, basil, oregano, salt, and pepper
5. Bring the whole mix to a boil and lower down the heat, simmer for 5-10 minutes until all veggies are tender
6. Add zucchini and simmer for 5 minutes more
7. Sever hot and enjoy!

Nutrition Values (Per Serving)

Calories: 22 , Carbohydrates: 5g , Protein: 1g

The "Main" Thai Soup

Serving: 4 , Prep Time: 10 minutes, Cook Time: 15 minutes

SmartPoints: 1

Ingredients

- 3 cups chicken stocks
- 1 tablespoon tom yum paste
- ½ garlic clove, chopped
- 3 stalks lemongrass, chopped
- 2 kaffir lime leaves
- 2 skinless and boneless chicken breasts, shredded
- 4 ounces mushrooms, sliced
- 1 tablespoon fish sauce
- 1 tablespoon lime juice
- 1 teaspoon green chile pepper, chopped
- 1 bunch coriander, chopped
- 1 bunch coriander, chopped
- 1 sprig fresh basil, chopped

Directions

1. Take a large sized saucepan and add chicken stock
2. Bring the mix to a boil
3. Stir in tom yum paste, garlic and cook for 2 minutes
4. Stir in lemongrass, kaffir lime leaves and simmer for 5 minutes over low heat
5. Add mushrooms, fish sauce, green chile, lime juice, pepper and keep cooking over medium heat until blended well
6. Remove the heat and serve warm with a garnish of coriander and basil
7. Enjoy!

Nutrition Values (Per Serving)

Calories: 71 , Fat: 1.8g, Protein: 10g, Carbohydrate: 5g,

Delicious Emmenthal Soup

Serving: 2 , Prep Time: 5 minutes , Cook Time: 5 minutes

SmartPoints: 1

Ingredients

- 2 cups cauliflower, cut into florets
- 1 potato, cubed
- 2 cups vegetable stock
- 3 tablespoons Emmenthal cheese, cubed
- 2 tablespoons fresh chives
- 1 tablespoon pumpkin seeds
- 1 pinch nutmeg
- 1 pinch cayenne pepper

Directions

1. Take a pot and add vegetable broth, place it over medium heat and allow it to heat up
2. Add potatoes and cauliflower and cook them until tender
3. Transfer the veggies to a blender and puree
4. Return the pureed mixture to the broth and stir well
5. Season the soup with cayenne, nutmeg, salt, and pepper
6. Add Emmenthal cheese, chives and stir
7. Garnish with pumpkin seed and enjoy!

Nutrition Values(Per Serving)

Calories: 351 , Fats: 14g , Carbs:28g , Fiber: 4g

Chicken and Carrot Stew

Serving: 4 , Prep Time: 15 minutes , Cook Time: 6 hours

SmartPoints: 3

Ingredients

- 4 boneless chicken breasts, cubed
- 3 cups of carrots, peeled and cubed
- 1 cup onion, chopped
- 1 cup tomatoes, chopped
- 1 teaspoon of dried thyme
- 2 cups of chicken broth
- 2 garlic cloves, minced
- Salt and pepper as needed

Directions

1. Add all of the listed ingredients to a Slow Cooker
2. Stir and close the lid
3. Cook for 6 hours
4. Serve hot and enjoy!

Nutrition Values (Per Serving)

Calories: 182 , Fat: 3g , Carbohydrates: 10g , Protein: 39g

Chapter 7 Fish and Seafood

Shrimp and Cilantro Meal

Serving: 4 , Prep Time: 10 minutes , Cook Time: 5 minutes

SmartPoints: 0

Ingredients

- 1 and ¾ pounds shrimp, deveined and peeled
- 2 tablespoons fresh lime juice
- ¼ teaspoon cloves, minced
- ½ teaspoon ground cumin
- 1 tablespoon olive oil
- 1 and ¼ cup fresh cilantro, chopped
- 1 teaspoon lime zest
- ½ teaspoon salt
- ¼ teaspoon pepper

Direction

1. Take a large sized bowl and add shrimp, cumin, garlic, lime juice, ginger and toss well
2. Take a large sized non-stick skillet and add oil, allow the oil to heat up over medium-high heat
3. Add shrimp mixture and Sauté for 4 minutes
4. Remove the heat and add cilantro, lime zest, salt, and pepper
5. Mix well and serve hot!

Nutrition Values (Per Serving)

Calories: 177 , Fat: 6g , Carbohydrates: 2g , Protein: 27g

Squid and Egg Meal

Serving: 4 , Prep Time: 15 minutes , Cook Time: 10 minutes

SmartPoints: 5

Ingredients

- 2 pounds squid, cleaned and cut into rings
- 2 eggs, beaten
- 2 teaspoon of olive oil
- ½ a yellow onion, sliced
- ½ a teaspoon of ground turmeric
- Salt as needed

Direction

1. Take a skillet and place it over medium-high heat
2. Add oil and allow the oil to heat up
3. Add onions and Sauté for 5 minutes
4. Add turmeric and squid rings, season with salt
5. Simmer over medium-low heat for 5 minutes
6. Add beaten eggs
7. Cook for an additional 3 minutes and serve immediately
8. Enjoy!

Nutrition Values (Per Serving)

Calories: 178 , Fat: 6g , Carbohydrates: 6g , Protein: 25g

The Original Dijon Fish

Serving: 2 , Prep Time: 3 minutes , Cook Time: 12 minutes

SmartPoints: 2

Ingredients

- 1 perch, flounder or sole fish florets
- 1 tablespoon Dijon mustard
- 1 and ½ teaspoon lemon juice
- 1 teaspoon low sodium Worcestershire sauce
- 2 tablespoons Italian seasoned bread crumbs
- 1 butter flavored cooking spray

Directions

1. Preheat your oven to 450 degrees Fahrenheit
2. Take an 11 x 7-inch baking dish and arrange your fillets carefully
3. Take a small sized bowl and add lemon juice, Worcestershire sauce, mustard and mix it well
4. Pour the mix over your fillet
5. Sprinkle a good amount of breadcrumbs
6. Bake for 12 minutes until fish flakes off easily
7. Cut the fillet in half portions and enjoy!

Nutrition Values (Per Serving)

Calories: 125 , Fat: 2g , Carbohydrates: 6g , Protein: 21g

Baked Zucchini Wrapped Fish

Serving: 2 , Prep Time: 15 minutes , Cook Time: 15 minutes

SmartPoints: 0

Ingredients

- 24-ounces cod fillets, skin removed
- 1 tablespoon of blackening spices
- 2 zucchinis, sliced lengthwise from to form ribbon
- ½ a tablespoon of olive oil

Directions

1. Season the fish fillets with blackening spice
2. Wrap each fish fillets with zucchini ribbons
3. Place fish on a plate
4. Take a skillet and place it over medium heat
5. Pour oil and allow the oil to heat up
6. Add wrapped fish to the skillet and cook each side for 4 minutes
7. Serve and enjoy!

Nutrition Values (Per Serving)

Calories: 397 , Fat: 23g , Carbohydrates: 2g , Protein: 46g

Spicy Baked Shrimp

Serving: 4 , Prep Time: 10 minutes , Cook Time: 25 minutes + 2-4 hours

Smart Points: 2

Ingredients

- ½ ounces large shrimp, peeled and deveined
- Cooking spray as needed
- 1 teaspoon low sodium soy sauce
- 1 teaspoon parsley
- ½ teaspoon olive oil
- ½ tablespoon honey
- 1 tablespoon lemon juice

Directions

1. Pre-heat your oven to 450 degrees F
2. Take a baking dish and grease it well
3. Mix in all the ingredients and toss
4. Transfer to oven and bake for 8 minutes until shrimp turn pink
5. Serve and enjoy!

Nutrition Values (Per Serving)

Calories: 321 , Fat: 9g , Carbohydrates: 44g , Protein: 22g

Asparagus Loaded Lobster Salad

Serving: 4 , Prep Time: 10 minutes , Cook Time: Nil

Smart Points: 5

Ingredients

- 8 ounces lobster, cooked and chopped
- 3 and ½ cups asparagus, chopped and steamed
- 2 tablespoon lemon juice
- 4 teaspoons extra virgin olive oil
- ¼ teaspoon kosher salt
- Pepper
- ½ cup cherry tomatoes halved
- 1 basil leaf, chopped
- 2 tablespoons red onion, diced

Directions

1. Whisk in lemon juice, salt, pepper in a bowl and mix with oil
2. Take a bowl and add rest of the ingredients
3. Toss well and pour dressing on top
4. Serve and enjoy!

Nutrition Values (Per Serving)

Calories: 247 , Fat: 10g , Carbohydrates: 14g , Protein: 27g

Spinach and Feta Stuffed Tilapia

Serving: 5, Prep Time: 10 minutes, Cook Time: 25 minutes

Smart Points: 6

Ingredients

- 16 ounces tilapia fillets
- Pinch of salt and pepper
- 1 egg beaten
- ½ cup part-skim ricotta cheese
- ½ cup crumbled feta cheese
- ½ cup bread crumbs
- 1 cup fresh spinach leaves, chopped
- ¼ teaspoon salt
- ¼ teaspoon pepper
- ¼ teaspoon dried thyme leaves
- 1 large lemon

Directions

1. Pre-heat your oven to 350 degrees F
2. Splash 2-quart heating dish with cooking shower, pat fish dry with paper towels and sprinkle salt and pepper
3. Take a bowl and blend in eggs and ricotta, until smooth
4. Add in feta, bread pieces, spinach, ¼ teaspoon salt, ¼ teaspoon dark pepper, thyme
5. Partition mixture between the fillet and carefully roll the fish, secure using a toothpick
6. Transfer to the heating dish (crease side down) and crush lemon juice on top
7. Cover and cook for 25 minutes, the stuffing should be ready
8. Enjoy!

Nutrition Values (Per Serving)

Calories: 181, Fat: 7g, Carbohydrates: 9g, Protein: 21g

Lemon and Garlic Scallops

Serving: 4, Prep Time: 10 minutes, Cook Time: 5 minutes

SmartPoints: 2

Ingredients

- 1 tablespoon olive oil
- 1 and ¼ pounds dried scallops
- 2 tablespoons all-purpose flour
- ¼ teaspoon salt
- 4-5 garlic cloves, minced
- 1 scallion, chopped
- 1 pinch of ground sage
- 1 lemon juice
- 2 tablespoons parsley, chopped

Direction

1. Take a non-stick skillet and place it over medium-high heat
2. Add oil and allow the oil to heat up
3. Take a medium sized bowl and add scallops alongside salt and flour
4. Place the scallops in the skillet and add scallions, garlic, and sage
5. Sauté for 3-4 minutes until they show an opaque texture
6. Stir in lemon juice and parsley
7. Remove heat and serve hot!

Nutrition Values (Per Serving)

Calories: 151 , Fat: 4g , Carbohydrates: 10g , Protein: 18g

Classic Tuna Salad

Serving: 4 , Prep Time: 10 minutes , Cook Time: Nil

SmartPoints: 1

Ingredients

- 12 ounces white tuna, in water
- ½ cup celery, diced
- 2 tablespoons fresh parsley, chopped
- 2 tablespoons low-calorie mayonnaise
- ½ teaspoon Dijon mustard
- ½ teaspoon salt
- ¼ teaspoon fresh ground black pepper

Direction

1. Take a medium sized bowl and add tuna, parsley, and celery
2. Mix well and add mayonnaise
3. Season with pepper and salt
4. Stir and add olives, relish, chopped pickle, onion and mix well
5. Serve and enjoy

Nutrition Values (Per Serving)

Calories: 137 , Fat: 5g , Carbohydrates: 1g , Protein: 20g

Shrimp Scampi

Serving: 4, Prep Time: 25 minutes, Cook Time: Nil

SmartPoints: 1

Ingredients

- 4 teaspoons olive oil
- 1 and ¼ pounds medium shrimp
- 6-8 garlic cloves, minced
- ½ cup low sodium chicken broth
- ½ cup dry white wine
- ¼ cup fresh lemon juice
- ¼ cup fresh parsley + 1 tablespoon extra, minced
- ¼ teaspoon salt
- ¼ teaspoon fresh ground pepper
- 4 slices lemon

Directions

1. Take a large sized bowl and place it over medium-high heat
2. Add oil and allow the oil to heat up
3. Add shrimp and cook for 2-3 minutes
4. Add garlic and cook for 30 seconds
5. Take a slotted spoon and transfer the cooked shrimp to a serving platter
6. Add broth, lemon juice, wine, ¼ cup of parsley, pepper, and salt to the skillet
7. Bring the whole mix to a boil
8. Keep boiling until the sauce has been reduced to half
9. Spoon the sauce over the cooked shrimp
10. Garnish with parsley and lemon
11. Serve and enjoy!

Nutrition Values (Per Serving)

Calories: 184, Fat: 6g, Carbohydrates: 6g, Protein: 15g

Chapter 8 Desserts

Beautiful Banana Custard

Serving: 3 , Prep Time: 10 minutes , Cook Time: 25 minutes

SmartPoints: 2

Ingredients

- 2 ripe bananas, peeled and mashed finely
- ½ a teaspoon of vanilla extract
- 14-ounce unsweetened almond milk
- 3 eggs

Directions

1. Pre-heat your oven to 350 degrees Fahrenheit
2. Grease 8 custard glasses lightly
3. Arrange the glasses in a large baking dish
4. Take a large bowl and mix all of the ingredients and mix them well until combined nicely
5. Divide the mixture evenly between the glasses
6. Pour water in the baking dish
7. Bake for 25 minutes
8. Take it out and serve
9. Enjoy!

Nutrition Values (Per Serving)

Calories: 59 , Fat: 2.4g , Carbohydrates: 7g , Protein: 3g

Carrot Ball Delight

Serving: 4 , Prep Time: 10 minutes , Cook Time: Nil

Smart Points: 2

Ingredients

- 6 Medjool dates pitted
- 1 carrot, finely grated
- ¼ cup of raw walnuts
- ¼ cup of unsweetened coconut, shredded
- 1 teaspoon of nutmeg
- 1/8 teaspoon of salt

Directions

1. Take a food processor and add dates, ¼ cup of grated carrots, salt coconut, nutmeg
2. Mix well and puree the mixture
3. Add the walnuts and remaining ¼ cup of carrots
4. Pulse the mixture until you have a chunky texture
5. Form balls using your hand and roll them up in coconut
6. Top with carrots and chill
7. Enjoy!

Nutrition Values (Per Serving)

Calories: 326 , Fat: 16g , Carbohydrates: 42g , Protein: 3g

Lovely Blueberry Pudding

Serving: 4 , Prep Time: 20 minutes , Cook Time: Nil

Smart Points: 0

Ingredients

- 2 cups of frozen blueberries
- 2 teaspoon of lime zest, grated freshly
- 20 drops of liquid stevia
- 2 small avocados, peeled, pitted and chopped
- ½ a teaspoon of fresh ginger, grated freshly
- 4 tablespoon of fresh lime juice
- 10 tablespoons of water

Directions

1. Add all of the listed ingredients to a blender (except blueberries) and pulse the mixture well
2. Transfer the mix into small serving bowls and chill the bowls
3. Serve with a topping of blueberries
4. Enjoy!

Nutrition Values (Per Serving)

Calories: 166 , Fat: 13g , Carbohydrates: 13g , Protein: 1.7g

Heart Warming vanilla Crepes

Serving: 3 , Prep Time: 5 minutes , Cook Time: 5 minutes

Smart Points: 6

Ingredients

- 2 whole eggs
- ½ tablespoon olive oil
- ½ teaspoon vanilla extract
- 1 tablespoon almond flour
- 1 tablespoon arrowroot powder
- ¼ teaspoon ground cinnamon
- Salt to taste

Directions

1. Take a bowl and mix in almond flour, salt, cinnamon, arrowroot powder, and mix
2. Beat eggs, vanilla together in another bowl
3. Add egg mix and flour mix and keep it on the side
4. Take a non-stick pan and place it over medium heat, add ¼ of mix and tilt well to coat the bottom in a thin layer
5. Cook for 1 minute each side
6. Repeat with remaining mixture and enjoy!

Nutrition Values (Per Serving)

Calories: 194 , Fat: 14g , Carbohydrates: 8g , Protein: 9g

Mesmerizing Ham Muffins

Serving: 4 , Prep Time: 5 minutes , Cook Time: 20 minutes

Smart Points: 6

Ingredients

- 4 ounces cooked ham, crumbled
- 4 whole eggs
- ½ cup red bell peppers, seeded and chopped
- 1 tablespoon water
- ½ cup onion, chopped
- Salt and pepper to taste

Directions

1. Pre-heat your oven to 360 degrees F
2. Grease 4 cups of a muffin tin
3. Take a bowl and beat in egg, water, salt and pepper
4. Beat well until combined
5. Add pepper, onions, ham and divide the mixture into muffin cups
6. Bake for 20 minutes
7. Serve and enjoy once done!

Nutrition Values (Per Serving)

Calories: 12 , Fat: 7g , Carbohydrates: 10g , Protein: 4g

Gentle Blackberry Crumble

Serving: 4 , Prep Time: 10 minutes , Cook Time: 45 minutes

Smart Points: 4

Ingredients

- ½ a cup of coconut flour
- ½ a cup of banana, peeled and mashed
- 6 tablespoons of water
- 3 cups of fresh blackberries
- ½ a cup of arrowroot flour
- 1 and a ½ teaspoon of baking soda
- 4 tablespoons of butter, melted
- 1 tablespoon of fresh lemon juice

Directions

1. Pre-heat your oven to 300 degrees F
2. Take a baking dish and grease it lightly
3. Take a bowl and mix all of the ingredients except blackberries, mix well
4. Place blackberries in the bottom of your baking dish and top with flour
5. Bake for 40 minutes
6. Serve and enjoy!

Nutrition Values (Per Serving)

Calories: 12 , Fat: 7g , Carbohydrates: 10g , Protein: 4g

Refreshing Watermelon Sorbet

Serving: 4 , Prep Time: 20 minutes + 20 hours chill time , Cook Time: Nil

Smart Points: 2

Ingredients

- 4 cups watermelons, seedless and chunked
- ¼ cup of superfine sugar
- 2 tablespoon of lime juice

Directions

1. Add the listed ingredients to a blender and puree
2. Transfer to a freezer container with a tight-fitting lid
3. Freeze the mix for about 4-6 hours until you have gelatin-like consistency
4. Puree the mix once again in batches and return to the container
5. Chill overnight
6. Allow the sorbet to stand for 5 minutes before serving and enjoy!

Nutrition Values (Per Serving)

Calories: 91 , Fat: 0g , Carbohydrates: 25g , Protein: 1g

Conclusion

I would like to thank you again for purchasing the book and taking the time to go through the book as well.

I do hope that this book has been helpful and you found the information contained within the scriptures useful!

Keep in mind that you are not only limited to the recipes provided in this book! Just go ahead and keep on exploring until you find the best Weight Watchers Freestyle regime that works for you!

Stay healthy and stay safe!

CPSIA information can be obtained
at www.ICGtesting.com
Printed in the USA
LVHW101526140121
676186LV00021B/480

9 781637 332238